A Comprehensive Guide to
Finding the Right Doctor
Tips from a Healthcare Credentialing Expert
Revised Edition

By Dilsa S. Bailey, CPMSM

A Comprehensive Guide to

Finding the Right Doctor

Tips from a Healthcare Credentialing Expert

Revised Edition

By Dilsa S. Bailey, CPMSM

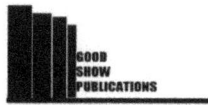

GOOD
SHOW
PUBLICATIONS

Dedication to the Health-Conscious Reader:

There is no way to fully express the amount of panic, uncertainty, and fear that is often attached to hearing your diagnosis for the first time. Even if we assume every doctor does their best, it doesn't mean that they are the best doctor for you. Encountering the good, the bad, and the in-between in healthcare providers throughout my career as a medical services professional working with hospitals and insurers, I want to share my insights to help you make an educated decision when choosing whom to trust with your life. Let me help ensure that once you have heard the words "the results were positive" or "your condition is not good," you know that the person treating you is helping you live the best quality of life you can at optimal health with your condition.

Yours truly,

Dilsa S. Bailey, CPMSM

What People Are Saying About This Book!

"Our health is our most valuable asset. Without it nothing else matters. The most important person for keeping you healthy is you. It is important we learn to build a collaborative relationship with the right healthcare team. This may seem like a daunting task but this book will guide you through the process of understanding how to determine if you're getting what you need from your health care providers. From the credentialing process for providers to links on how to find information about your providers, this book covers it all. The included forms guide you in putting together your healthcare team and ensure you are prepared with the right providers before you have a health crisis. This is a must read for everyone".

Marie Giarniero, BSN, MS, RN, CNOR

∞

"Reading **A Comprehensive Guide to Finding the Right Doctor** by Dilsa Bailey is like sitting down with a friend and talking about health. With a conversational style that helps clear the murkiness of the world of healthcare, Ms. Bailey provides excellent explanations of medical terms that we routinely hear but may not really know. She provides step-by-step advice for picking out doctors, with great tips on what to consider. As a Caregiver Consultant, I especially appreciated the hands-on tools in her appendix, such as the Physician Directory and Medication History form. This is information I would encourage all adults (and any caregivers) to consider. I think this book will be particularly helpful for anyone making changes in their life, whether you are moving, having health changes or aging, her clear explanations into the background of healthcare and how to assess your health care team can provide extra confidence in choosing your doctor."

Jessica Knopf Dugan (Caregiver Consultant)

"This is a book full of information that many of us should know, but unfortunately don't, when it comes to understanding and navigating the complicated world of finding quality healthcare providers. This book can also serve as a great reference tool to assist with gaining a better understanding of terms commonly used when seeking various medical treatments or services."

Frank Jones, LMFT (Licensed Marriage and Family Therapist)

∞

"I have been pretty blessed with finding the right healthcare professionals on my path to better health. I also understand there are too many instances it may not be the case and finding the right doctor care is very challenging. Ms. Bailey's guide to finding the right doctor is a great resource for not just asking those general questions to navigate your personal health decisions, but also having more specific information at your fingertips".

Vivian H. (Cancer Survivor)

Contents

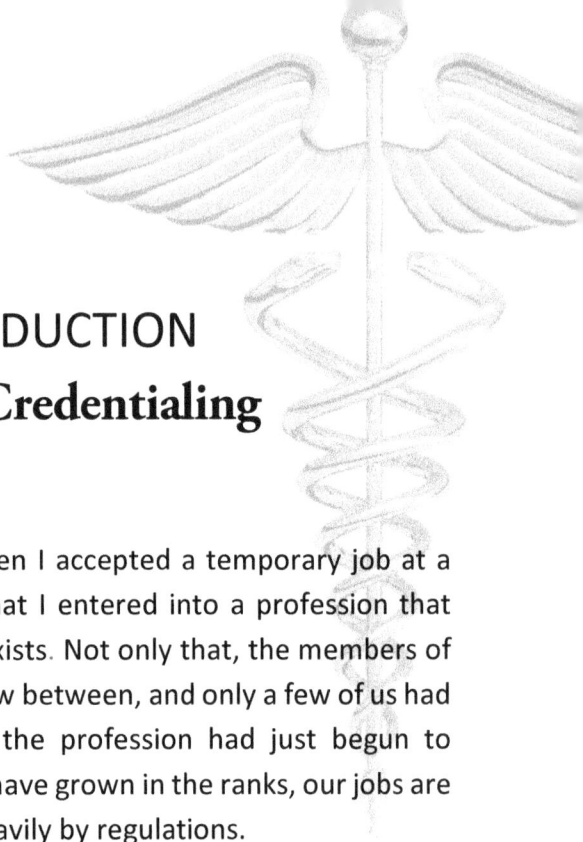

INTRODUCTION
What is Credentialing

Little did I know that when I accepted a temporary job at a hospital 30 years ago that I entered into a profession that very few people know exists. Not only that, the members of our profession were far and few between, and only a few of us had the necessary skills because the profession had just begun to evolve. Though, our numbers have grown in the ranks, our jobs are very specialized and driven heavily by regulations.

What does this mean? The stronger your expertise, the more sought after you are, with an emphasis on *expertise*. Not only do you have to perform the little details, you have to know what's relevant to patient care. And that's why this book exists: to help you identify what's relevant to you and to support your efforts to seek the best health care. Remember, it almost always starts with you, setting aside emergent and urgent events. We need this information to help us navigate the waters of healthcare that is ever changing, especially when we are dealing with pandemics such as the COVID-19 Virus in 2020-2022 and, maybe, by the time the third revision of this book is necessary, through 2023. Let's hope not.

So, what am I? What do I do that can help you choose the right health care provider? I am a medical services professional specializing in **credentialing** healthcare providers.

To perform credentialing, it is my responsibility to make sure that the practitioners who provide healthcare to patients in hospitals or to members of healthcare plans are qualified and competent to do so. The credentialing specialist ensures that the doctor on staff at the hospital can provide the quality of care that has been benchmarked by the healthcare organization. It is that organization's responsibility to make sure the doctor's credentials are indeed real and that he or she is really an advanced healthcare professional.

The act of credentialing ensures that the medical doctors, podiatrists, oral surgeons, nurse practitioners, chiropractors, and other advanced degree healthcare professionals are who they say they are and can do what they say they can do. It is a tedious job, but the mantra in our profession is this: "There is no other master but the patient." It is all about you.

Usually, the job involves long hours combing through documents, gathering and analyzing data, and then presenting the findings to a professional panel of peers comprised of medical doctors and advanced healthcare professionals. These panels or committees review these documents from a skilled, clinical perspective to determine if the applicants for hospital staff membership or managed care participation pass the organization's quality benchmark. Each organization — whether it is a hospital or a managed care company — has a set of policies or bylaws that outlines the skill set and requirements for each provider. Before your doctor can be granted permission to work with either of these organizations, they must meet those requirements.

In addition to meeting an organization's basic requirements, there are several other sets of rules that require the organization to establish policies and procedures or bylaws. Those rules are passed down from the federal government's Centers for Medicare and Medicaid Services (CMS) and accrediting agencies such as The Joint Commission (TJC) or the National Committee for Quality Assurance (NCQA).

Now, to answer the question, *what is credentialing?*

Credentialing is the process of selecting and evaluating practitioners who provide health care services. How do we do that? Medical services professionals, usually called credentialing specialists, collect data to see if the healthcare provider meets established requirements. Hospital and health plan requirements vary slightly, but here are the basics that must be collected and verified:

— Active License to practice in their practicing state. This includes those telehealth professionals that may be treating you from a different state over the internet or by telephone.

— Federal Drug Enforcement Administration's registrations for the state where the doctor practices; or state-controlled substances registrations determining the level of narcotic prescriptions that can be written.

— Evidence of education and training, such as medical schools, residencies and fellowships, and board certifications, or other professional certifications required to practice.

— Malpractice coverage limits and coverage dates.

— Hospital affiliations, admitting privileges for diagnoses, treatments, or surgical procedures that are congruent with training and experience or arrangements to provide hospital care.

— National Practitioner Data Bank (NPDB) report. The NPDB is a federal database that requires licensing agencies to report adverse or disciplinary actions; liability insurance companies to report any paid judgments or settlements made by the insurer; or hospitals and healthcare organizations to report any loss of privileges or rights to treat patients.

— Office of Inspector General (OIG), Medicare/Medicaid Opt-Out, System for Award Management (SAM) formerly the Excluded Parties List Service (EPLS) reports, or State Exclusions Lists. The credentialing specialist will determine if a provider can accept Medicare or Medicaid funds. Reasons that exclude them from acceptance of payments of healthcare funds include fraud and abuse (OIG), voluntary opt-outs from participating in Medicare and Medicaid programs; or, for a variety of reasons, an inability to contract with different state or federal government.

— Criminal Background checks are more commonly performed by hospitals than managed care organizations.

Other review and collection activity resides usually outside of the credentialing track but is included in the review process when your doctor or provider undergoes a review cycle. That activity is called a **quality review**. A quality review looks closer at practice patterns and a continued ability to function under the privileges granted in a hospital setting and, from a different perspective, practice patterns and the continued ability to participate on a network panel in a health plan setting.

Now that you are familiar with the responsibilities of a credentialing professional to make sure the doctors practicing in hospital and managed care (health plan) settings can effectively provide you with competent healthcare, what is it that **you** can do to determine if one of those doctors can meet your specific needs? In the next chapters, let's review the basic credentialing steps you can perform on your behalf. Then we can cover the dynamics of the type of relationship you desire with your physician, and who would be your best fit.

CHAPTER 1
What Can You Find Out About Your Doctor?

I had lived in Philadelphia for 13 years prior to my move to Atlanta, leaving behind a network of friends, family, and other support, including my doctors. But after the move, I had to look for a new gynecologist, a new primary care physician, a new dentist, and a new pediatrician. Although I had been in the credentialing field for several years prior to my move, choosing a doctor was still a crap shoot, which, I hate to tell you, it is for everyone. This book will give you a little more ammunition toward a successful relationship and I will walk you through the basic information so you can discover for yourself. However, *recommendations from friends, colleagues, and reputable reviewing sites are still going to be key*. I will mention those sites later in this book.

Licensing

First, let's look at **licensing**. Most state licensing agencies have a free website with a page usually called **license lookup** or **license verification**. Many of these states' medical licensing agencies are called **medical boards**. Some names of these agencies differ though, e.g., Washington Medical Commission. See **RESOURCES** for a listing of or link to all the licensing boards. You should be able to find your provider by name, specialty, and location.

So, what information will you get?

The site will tell you when the license was issued, when it will expire, and whether it's active. Most importantly, it will tell you if there are any disciplinary actions taken against your physician. Sometimes you will find an innocuous fine for not taking the necessary number of Continuing Medical Education (CME's) courses during a certain timeframe to maintain their licenses (usually discovered during a random state audit). Sometimes you may find that a provider was mandated to take a few extra CMEs in a certain area, such as overprescribing or addressing issues with medical records. The reasons will vary.

Some actions may make you take a pause before going forward. Board actions can be serious, and most states will have them available for your review right there with the verification of licensure. **CAUTION:** When reading these, remember that your physician or potential physician is human and if it is someone you already know, maybe you can get a feel for the context and timeframe for the actions. Or, if it's public, ask for an explanation if it is something that concerns you. I am providing this information to you *as a tool though and not as a weapon unless you plan to litigate. My advice is if you don't like what you find, find another doctor.*

Another item of interest is that most medical boards post their disciplinary actions on a monthly basis. It is not something you would want to monitor, but your health plan or hospital is required to do so within 30 days of the information's release.

Education and Training
(including Board Certification)

State medical licensure boards are extremely consumer friendly. They provide Physician Profiles because they believe you should know your doctor and will give you the information you need directly from the doctor. Doctors complete these questionnaires when they apply for a license, and they have to update their profiles regularly. Physician Profiles list the medical schools they attended, the residency programs, and the fellowships. Licensing agencies verify the education and training of these individuals prior to issuing a license, so a profile is usually accurate. But the accuracy of the overall profile may depend on whether the doctor completed it or had an office staff member do so. Errors happen. However, the education and training should be correct as it has been verified.

Another way to determine if the provider is qualified and competent in his specialty is to check for **board certification**. Not to scare you, but some people are better at testing than others. However, board certification is a great benchmark to assess your provider's skillset. The certifying board institutions that are members of the American Board of Medical Specialties (ABMS) are starting to require continuous education for ongoing maintenance of certification to ensure that the providers continually demonstrate competence. Prior to being eligible to take a board, a physician must have adequate education and training in that specialty area. The most common primary specialties include general surgery, internal medicine, pediatrics, obstetrics and gynecology, radiology, emergency medicine, orthopedics, and anesthesiology. Visit the ABMS Website; it will list the primary specialties and their subspecialties.

Subspecialties require additional focused training and experience. For instance, **internal medicine** is a primary specialty and cardiovascular disease would be a subspecialty. Physicians would pursue a board certification in internal medicine first, and then as their practice and training are more specialized in cardiovascular disease, they would pursue board certification for that. Their additional training may have been called a fellowship giving them more detailed and more cardiovascular driven experience. Board certification is the highest level of competency a physician can attain and to what all physicians and advanced practitioners aspire.

Hospital Affiliations

Managed care organizations (MCO), your health plan, contract with hospitals in what is called a *participating network*. They would prefer their network providers or physicians admit to those participating hospitals. Even Medicare looks at whether a physician has admitting privileges at a hospital. If no privileges, they look for an arrangement to treat their patients in a hospital setting. Hospitals also query other hospitals to determine if their physicians are undergoing quality review activities elsewhere, i.e., disciplinary actions or the inability to practice certain procedures. At any rate, hospital privileges (what one can and cannot do in a hospital setting) is an important aspect as a benchmark of competency. For the patient, it is important to know where the doctor would want to admit you, and whether that doctor would be able to treat you in that setting.

In today's practice environment, many primary care physicians are opting out of hospital privileges. Like many of us, they would like to have some down time and a regularly scheduled life. If they see their patients who have been admitted to a hospital, they will have less time to practice. Patients in a hospital must be *seen*, meaning their doctors must perform rounds.

Rounds entail walking through the hospital, checking charts, examining and chatting with patients, or meeting with staff tracking the patient, and following up with paperwork (medical record keeping, billing, etc.). It is a very time-consuming job, and that is why most hospitals employ various types of physicians, such as internists, neurologists (specializing in stroke victims), neonatologists, and intensivists (specializing in critical care medicine) to staff their floors 24 hours per day. These employed physicians are called *hospitalists*. This allows the individual primary care physician to send a patient to a hospital, and to be kept abreast of their patients' treatments through medical records supplied by those hospitalists. If a patient is admitted for more specialized treatment, it is usually the doctor on call assigned to that specialty who will track them, or the doctor who was already a part of the treatment, admitting, or referral process.

What does all of this mean for you?
Choose a hospital or hospital system where you wish to be treated, whether because it is close to your home or that it provides the specialty care your health dictates. **Then, think about choosing your doctor.** Hospitals usually have directories on their

websites with a section for each specialty type. These directories are a good place to start when searching for a physician. You can also familiarize yourself with the type of hospital services provided there as well. Then what? Determine if the physician you are choosing has chosen to participate in your health plan's network, whether its Blue Cross, Aetna, and others and whether it's their HMO, PPO, or Indemnity product. Not all practitioners sign up for all products offered by the health plan.

Accept Medicaid or Medicare?

The agencies I mentioned previously are just a few clicks away, if you need a physician that accepts either Medicare or Medicaid. Or it can be as simple as calling the doctor's office or checking the doctor's website. Most physicians will list the plans they accept, including Medicare or Medicaid. But, if you want to do your own credentialing, you can go to the Office of Inspector General's website or the System for Award Management's website, or to one of the regional websites for opt-out (See **RESOURCES**). Honestly, it is easier for the general public to just check with the doctor's office or to go directly to the Medicare site.

Criminal Activity

Doctors are human and have the same mental and moral afflictions as do the general public. Some make simple mistakes: drinking too much in college and getting caught; or, major mistakes, such as a hit and run while under the influence; some actions are much, much worse. There are doctors who fall in love with their patients and others who have been known for sexual assaults. But most *doctors are upright citizens like the rest of us and only want to provide quality care to their patients while providing a decent income for their families.* If the healthcare organization's credentialing review is not enough for you, there are so many options to conduct your own criminal background search. It is not unlike doing a search on anyone else in the world; you can browse through your state or county's criminal websites or use an Internet search company like Sentry Link. How invasive you want to be into your doctor's life or practice should be totally dependent on any concerns you may have in your individual treatment. If it's something egregious, report it to your local law enforcement. If you don't feel safe, don't go back. Find another doctor.

Quality of Care

Healthcare organizations continuously monitor their doctors and practitioners providing direct care to their patients. The process is called many things: peer review processes, quality review, ongoing professional practice evaluations, focused professional practice evaluations, the CMS STARS rating, and more. These evaluations are based on practice activity, medical records reviews, complaints, grievances, appeals, utilization of resources provided by the healthcare organization, and performance. The details of these are not accessible to the public, but the website, Health Grades can give you a snapshot of the hospital and the doctor.

Recommendations

These days, finding a doctor is becoming a bit easier with recommendations on websites such as Suggest A Doctor or Healthcare Reviews. Query Google or any web browser and you will find many, many more options. Your friends and neighbors are a great source of recommendations: Word of mouth of who is good and who is bad never fails. *However, remember you and your friends may differ on the characteristics of a great doctor. Don't forget to ask what the basis is for their recommendations.*

Personally Satisfied?

Caution: Don't go overboard and probe too much. You don't need to know every detail of your doctor's life. There have been many days when I felt guilty of voyeurism for the things we make these professionals divulge. All you need to know is that they will provide you with the best care possible; they will be reliable and dependable when they are most needed; and they will meet your healthcare needs to the best of their ability based on their education, training, and experience.

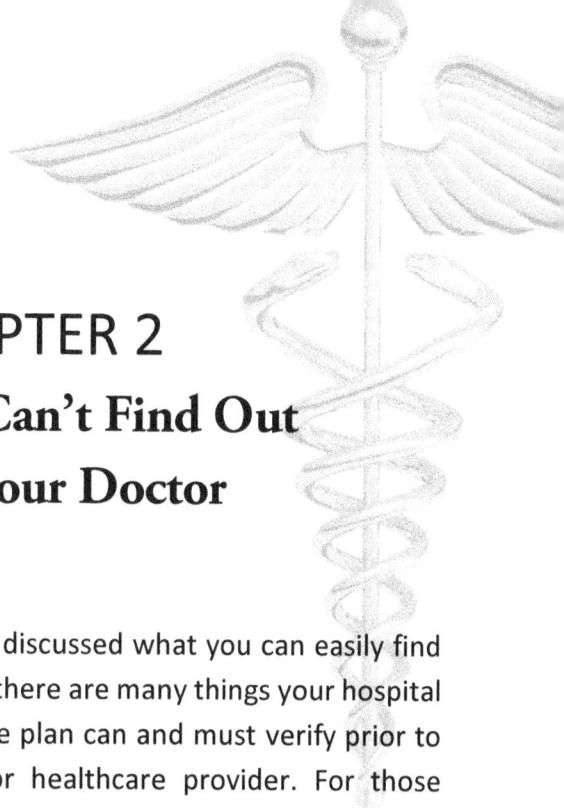

CHAPTER 2
What You Can't Find Out About Your Doctor

I n the previous chapter, we discussed what you can easily find out about your doctor. But there are many things your hospital of choice or your healthcare plan can and must verify prior to affiliation with your doctor or healthcare provider. For those organizations to go through the credentialing or verification process, the doctor must authorize them to do so by providing an application and the supporting documentation they need to meet the healthcare organization's requirements. Below are a few items that the healthcare organization reviews that you, as a member of the general public, would <u>not</u> have access to.

Ability to Prescribe Medications

The provider's ability to prescribe — including narcotic drug types — is off limits to you. The Drug Enforcement Administration (DEA) registration number and its schedules are protected to prohibit use by those not competent to prescribe and to prohibit criminal activity. Prescribing pain medications or other addictive medications are a source of the steadily growing culture of prescription medicine abuse. Pain management clinics have popped up around the country and are providing a steady flow of income for criminals preying on those addicted to prescription medications. That is why your doctor's staff should not be writing you a prescription on a pre-signed prescription pad. Your doctors should electronically prescribe directly to your pharmacy. No one should be prescribing unless they are authorized. In most states, nurse practitioners and physician assistants, in addition to your doctors, dentists, or podiatrists, can prescribe.

National Practitioner Data Bank

The doctor's report on the National Practitioner Data Bank (NPDB) is not available to the public. The Healthcare Quality Improvement Act of 1986 was responsible for the creation of the National Practitioner Data Bank. This data bank is a clearinghouse of state licensure actions, malpractice settlements, and issues of quality of care reported by healthcare organizations. Essentially, the purpose of this clearinghouse is to protect patients from unfit practitioners who may drift from place to place staying under the radar.

The NPDB makes it an easier process to find out if any adverse actions or sanctions have been imposed upon the practitioner, no matter where he practices in the United States. In addition to reports from healthcare organizations, the practitioner can self-report or to comment on any reports made related to his or her adverse actions. Healthcare organizations can not only report adverse actions but can determine if any negative practice trends have occurred before a doctor is approved for affiliation with their organization. And the doctor's comments can contribute to their final decisions.

Quality Review

Quality Review data collected by healthcare organizations are protected under state and federal peer review statutes. You won't be able to get your doctor's report card in these areas. The type of information collected helps these organizations determine, for instance, if a surgeon can still perform specific procedures. Perhaps, a general surgeon (let's call this surgeon George) has never performed bariatric surgery before and would not have the experience to do so. The hospital will not grant George those privileges if he applies for that. However, another scenario could be is that he does have the experience but has had a series of bad outcomes. Those privileges to perform that type of surgery may be removed, or George may be required to be proctored, or overseen, by another doctor with experience under review.

Healthcare organizations score such things as how long a patient is kept in a hospital; how many consults are requested and if they are related to the patient's condition; whether the patient acquires an infection in the hospital under the doctor's care; the average outcome of patients with a specific condition; and more. As a potential patient looking for decisive data, you would not be able to request or acquire this information. But rest assured, healthcare organizations are looking at that data more and more closely to meet their accreditation standards, to meet federal and state guidelines, and to make certain they are able to provide the best healthcare for their patients or members.

Why Would You Want to Know About Your Doctor?

Some people may think finding out details about your doctor is equivalent to snooping on your next-door neighbor. But your next-door neighbor won't routinely help you make decisions related to your health. Your doctor's ability to diagnose or treat your health concerns may be crucial to the length of your life as well as its quality.

Here are a few good and bad examples that have affected the lives of patients:

THE BAD

1) A man from Austell, Georgia, was arrested on August 24, 2012, for stealing a physician's identity and practicing medicine in South Carolina. For a year, he treated more than 500 patients using false documents to affiliate with a physician-recruiting agency and primary care centers for seniors.

2) In San Francisco, another man practiced as a dermatologist without training and without a license harming as many as nine patients in the process, as reported by California Watch.

3) Here is a familiar name for you: Conrad Murray overprescribed medications for music popstar, Michael Jackson. His negligence, most likely motivated by financial difficulties, led to Mr. Jackson's death.

4) Pain management clinics or pill mills are running rampant and under great scrutiny from the Drug Enforcement Administration, your local state bureaus of investigation, and medical licensing boards. Physicians prescribing medications without performing a history or physical, or any type of examination are being cited for overprescribing, especially to those addicted to prescription medications. Not only that, some physicians are also stooping low enough to prescribe a one-month supply of generic, immediate-release oxycodone-hydrochloride to anyone who walks into their offices, no matter how many times the addict requests a prescription, thus creating the need to scrutinize pharmacies as well. Two CVS stores in Florida near Orlando lost their controlled substance licenses because of indiscriminate dispensing of pain medications.

5) A case in the State of Washington details an anesthesiologist's addiction to Demerol, which was discovered after he participated in a surgery that rendered the patient in a vegetative state.

6) A Washington hospital began an investigation into an anesthesiologist. His patients were waking up in excessive pain though more than enough Fetanyl had been ordered. The doctor had been helping himself to the pain medication. According to a Minnesota Medicine article in February 2010, studies show "the rate of addiction among practicing physicians is estimated to be between 10% and 12%, the same as or slightly higher than the rate in the general population. Although alcohol is the primary

13

problem in nearly half of all cases, physicians are more likely than others to abuse prescribed medications."

7) A more common scenario: The patient has a persistent ache, a persistent pain, or a persistent condition and the doctor generalizes it, dropping it into the "benign symptom" bucket of a non-threatening condition. The diagnosis proves wrong, or worse yet, the condition becomes worse; the doctors are stumped and unable to diagnose or treat the condition.

8) What about one of the most known cases of Christopher Duntsch, more popularly known as Dr. Death? He had graduated from a residency without fully completing the program. As a result, this individual with a charming personality and grandiose ego permanently maimed and killed his patients over several years before he was finally stopped. Unfortunately, the tips in this book may not have protected you in this case. He was well-protected, and no one reported him until the situation became obviously dire.

What could be the problem with your provider?

After many opinions and still no decisive diagnosis, it is that unique situation *that may not be so unique to you*. Only time will tell. On the other hand, it could be that the one doctor you are relying on for the right diagnosis has skills that are not current. You may be encountering a competency problem. Competency is not only an issue with diagnosis; it is even more dangerous when the competency issue involves surgery. You could be dealing with an impaired physician, an unprepared physician, or an outdated physician.

THE GOOD

1) Recently, I heard a story about a man who had a persistent headache. After many doctor visits and tests of various kinds, the source of the headache remained a mystery. This man knew his body, knew something was wrong, and so kept returning to the doctors for help. Finally, one doctor sat down with him to review the films from the last battery of tests and to show the man nothing was there to be concerned with but, as the doctor detailed his findings, one little irregularity in the man's brain was discovered. The man's persistence saved his life, and his doctor's competency in recognizing the miniscule irregularity contributed. It was a team effort led by the patient who persisted because he knew something was wrong and he was not going to stop until it was found.

2) Early detection of cancer or other life-threatening diseases occur every day. Mammograms, pap smears, and tests of all kinds are reviewed and interpreted by competent doctors who identify the risk and expedite treatment to save lives.

3) The obstetrician may deliver a premature baby and then hand it over to a capable neonatologist who keeps the baby alive and well until it can go home with its mother with

every expectation of living a full and normal life. That happens every day.

4) Transplant teams successfully remove organs from a donor, and coordinating teams take the transported organs and successfully implant them into another body.

5) Everyone strives for a healthy, happy life. Doctors became doctors to help us achieve that, and so the type of credentialing information you *need* to know about your doctor should include:
   a. Licensure issues
   b. Training and experience related to the conditions for which you would be treated.
   c. Hospital or healthcare plan affiliations.

Now That You Know …

Now that you know what you can and cannot find out, what are the next steps? In the next chapter, we will discuss what it is you are looking for that will make you happy with your choice.

CHAPTER 3
Characteristics of
Your Favorite Doctor

Have you ever left the doctor's office a little peeved? You wondered if that doctor has heard a word you said. When I first moved to Atlanta, a co-worker referred me to a large group practice. Since this group practice was affiliated with a large academic institution that, in a few years, would employ me, I expected upscale service. *Wrong!* I was scheduled with one of the rudest human beings I had ever met. I don't think he heard one word of my concern. He was in a hurry, and everything I described about my condition was obviously frivolous to him. Did I go back? Of course, not! *So, what was the problem?*

Look for these characteristics in a doctor:

- *Does the doctor listen?*
- *Is the doctor respectful?*
- *Is the doctor open and honest with you?*

PERSONAL CHARACTERISTICS

Listen. In my case, did he *really* listen to me? No. And, when he did listen, he dismissed me. Now, I am not going to say he was wrong in his diagnosis; it was just the way he communicated it. I wasn't sure if he fully understood what I was saying. And I am a communicator. I will let you know what I want you to know as clearly as I possibly can and be persistent about it.

Some people, especially the elderly, may not communicate as clearly or are afraid to continue to impress upon the doctor their concerns because, well, *they're the doctor*. Forget that! The doctor is a human being who has been trained to provide a very specialized service. We all respect that, but they should, and most do, respect us, too.

Remember that. Tell the doctor what you need the doctor to know. Write it out if you don't think you will remember all the symptoms or concerns. Make a list. Give it to your doctor. So listening should be high on your priority list of characteristics. **Your doctor should be listening to your concerns, and actually repeating them back to you to ensure both of you are communicating clearly.**

Respect. Respect is up there next to listening. As I mentioned earlier, the doctor I saw had his head so far in the clouds, he didn't give me the respect I deserved. As a result, he lost a patient for himself, his group, and his healthcare organization. Years later, someone referred me to a colleague in his same practice, and I fell in love with her. She was my primary care physician (PCP) for over twelve years before she decided to become an administrator at her organization. She not only listened to me but treated me with respect. Sometimes, we giggled over my health concerns because I can be a bit of a hypochondriac. But I never felt bad about expressing my concerns, or even worse, felt afraid to express them. You should always feel that you can be open with your doctor. You should expect eye contact and the truth. Some doctors and patients develop authoritarian and subordinate relationships. Don't accept that. You are neither a child nor an unimportant voice in your own health decisions. And by the way, I have a great relationship with my current PCP.

Honest and open. Do you feel as if your doctor is hiding something? If that is your gut instinct, go with it and run out of the door. **Example:** A surgeon wants to operate on you. **Ask them:**

— *How many procedures of that type-have they performed?*

— *Are there complications or risks? If so, have they encountered any? If the answer is yes, ask how many?*

— *What is their success rate? You have a right to know. If they don't want you to know, that may not be a good thing.*

Find a surgeon who is not hiding their success or failure rate. On the flip side, some doctors may be hesitant to give their patients a whole diagnosis thinking the patient is not up to the news. That's not a good practice either. To promote better health or fix the problem, you need to know the whole truth. Shy away from doctors who are unable to be honest for any reason.

DOCTOR'S OFFICE CHARACTERISTICS

Look for these characteristics in a doctor's office:

— *How long do you have to wait for an appointment?*

— *How long is the wait in the waiting room?*

— *Who will be treating you — doctor, physician's assistant, or nurse practitioner?*

- *Is the lab work done inside or outside the office? How about X-rays?*
- *Is the office clean?*
- *Is the bathroom clean?*
- *Is the office easily accessible? Is it on the second floor without an elevator access?*

Availability. After determining if the doctor accepts my insurance, I look for **availability**: How long does it take for me to get an appointment? How long does it take their staff to answer the phone, if I need to get into the doctor's office? In my profession, I have called offices whose phones rang forever, and I have often wondered how that practice survives. Who is going to return my calls, the doctor or the doctor's nurse? Go ahead, ask the question when you call the office. Your insurance company will tell you if they are accepting new patients, the hours, the location, etc. But it's the representative answering the phone who will schedule your appointment. Ask how far out will you have to schedule your annual physical? If it is a condition that needs immediate treatment, how is it handled? The representative can give you a feel for the professional manner of the office.

The waiting room. This one has made me change doctors over the years. How long will I be in and how well will I get to know the other patients in the **waiting room**? Is there a sick area, especially in the pediatrician's office? Does your doctor overbook? Your time is just as valuable to you as the doctor's is to him or her. Ask the office representative what the average waiting time is. Doctors who are specialists, such as a surgeon or an OB/Gyn, get called to the hospital in emergencies and their schedules may occasionally run over. However, that is no excuse. It is called *covering physicians.* Will someone else be available if your doctor is still in the hospital treating other patients?

A good sign that the wait is not excessive is when you are required to arrive 15 minutes early for your appointment so that you can get all the necessary paperwork and co-pays out of the way. This gives you the impression of a well-oiled machine to get you in and out of the door quickly and without too much exposure to your fellow patients who may be carrying the latest bug.

Treating professional. Is there a doctor in the house? Who will be *treating* you in the doctor's office? Will you be seeing the doctor, nurse practitioner, or physician assistant? In today's health care environment, nurse practitioners and physician assistants are treating patients. For instance, you can go to a CVS Minute Clinic or a Walgreen's for routine illnesses like the flu, strep, and pink eye, etc. You can just walk-in, get treated, get the prescription, and be on your merry way. A nurse practitioner provides those services there and may be providing those services in your doctor's office as well. Ask the question, does your doctor employ those individuals and will they be treating you? This is not a reason <u>not</u> to choose a doctor; the nurse practitioner or physician assistant is supervised by the doctor who will be confirming their employees' treatment and diagnoses. You just want to be aware of the level of the professional who will be treating or examining you. FYI: The non-physician is required by most state laws to identify their profession before treating you. "Hi, I am Sam, nurse practitioner."

Lab work and X-rays. Are they performed onsite, or will you be referred to another location? Not every doctor's office is fully equipped with an X-ray machine, but lab work onsite is a plus. You could get your results in a shorter turnaround time, maybe not. Ask.

Cleanliness of space should be a requirement. The last thing I want to do is stare at a dirty or stained carpet, tattered chairs squeezed together so tightly one is trying to pop out of formation, and coffee-stained magazines tossed wildly about the waiting room. You don't want to see anything that is not pristine in the examining room, either. Examining tools should come right out of the packages used to store them after cleaning. The examining table should have been wiped down and a clean roll of paper put into place. Your healthcare providers, whether doctor, nurse, or other staff, must wash their hands before touching you. Expect nothing less.

OUT-OF-OFFICE CONSIDERATIONS

If you did not start your doctor search from an online hospital directory or the health plan directory, consider a future hospital stay. In which **hospital** would you prefer to be treated? Ask which hospital the doctor is with or the hospital to where he or she refers patients. Ask: Will the doctor be treating you in the hospital or a **hospitalist group**? Is it in your neighborhood, close to you and family, or is it too far away for access? Definitely something you need to consider.

Coordination of care is another consideration. Does your doctor utilize electronic medical records? Are those medical records shared with the hospital you would be staying in or with the consultant or specialist you would be referred to? Coordination of care is important because a conflict in treatment or prescriptions could occur. One doctor's prescription may cause an adverse reaction with another doctor's prescription. One recommended treatment could cause injury to another part of the body being treated for something else.

If your doctors or organizations are not talking to each other, you need to make sure you are talking to them all. A referral team or group affiliations help to promote coordination of care. But, the responsibility lies upon you as well. Take a list of your prescriptions and give each doctor your whole history, not bits and pieces.

Always expect professionalism from the staff. Whether clinical or non-clinical, from the receptionist to the phlebotomist, the doctor's staff is a reflection of him or her. You should be greeted, acknowledged, and treated with respect. You should expect the doctor to receive your messages, and the staff should relay your messages promptly.

Keep these characteristics in mind. Expect the best and receive the best, whether you are paying cash, using Medicaid or Medicare, or have commercial insurance. All patients are equal, but like all professions, all doctors are not. And like any other service provider, they should earn your hard-earned dollars no matter their source. Every aspect of the office reflects on your doctor and the type of services he or she provides, including the staff who greets you at the receptionist desk. Every aspect of their office, human and nonhuman, makes a difference in the care you receive.

Say NO to disparity.

Whether you want to believe it or not, there is disparity in our healthcare system. The most obvious factors are race and economic status. African Americans are statistically higher at being mistreated, ignored, or denied access to medical care. But the disparity does not end there, nor does it start there. First of all, medicine is a business, a foundational structure that thrives on its success to generate income. At times, learning how to generate that income by experimenting or researching involved using marginalization, racism, and capitalism as human factors. But you as an individual working with your healthcare provider as an individual can help reduce the continued incidents of disparity. It's going to take a lot more on the systemic level. But one-on-one communication is the basis for a start to reduce or eliminate this pandemic.

Keep in mind, that dependent on how your healthcare provider was raised, and to whom they were exposed throughout their lives will determine how open they are with you about the care you need. This is called *implicit bias*. Some may skip telling you all the details because, one, they may automatically assume you don't understand. Secondly, they may automatically assume that, if you did understand, you wouldn't do anything to change your behavior or habits to make your condition better. And lastly, they may automatically assume if you are uninsured or partially insured, that you couldn't do anything financially to help yourself anyway. Yes, these biased mindsets mostly affect African Americans. But don't fool yourself. If you are economically marginalized, speak broken English, come from another country, come from the inner city, or even grew up in the rural South (speaking with an accent outside the South), those to whom your doctor has been exposed to during their life and training will automatically paint a picture of who they think you are. That's why you have to step up, talk freely and, if you can't communicate effectively, take someone with you. Get an advocate. One of the best ways to stop disparity is to let your provider know you are human.

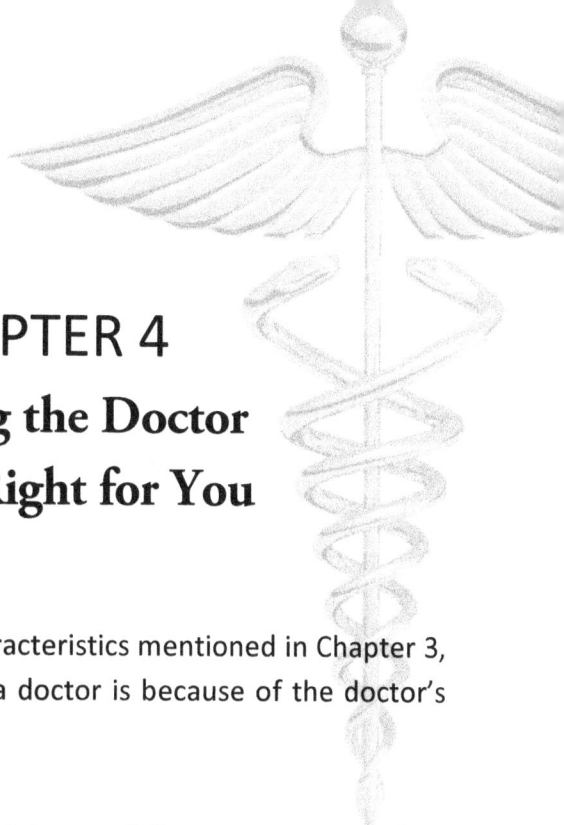

CHAPTER 4
Choosing the Doctor Who Is Right for You

K eeping in mind the characteristics mentioned in Chapter 3, one reason to choose a doctor is because of the doctor's specialty.

How do you know what type of doctor to go see?

Some health plan products let you self-refer instead of waiting for a referral from your primary care physician.

- – *Would you know who to choose?*
- – *When your PCP writes up a referral for you to see a specialist, are you clear on what the specialist does?*

Here are a few short descriptions on different specialties to help you choose a doctor that is right for you as published by the American Board of Internal Medicine and the American Board of Surgery. For further detail on all specialties and subspecialties, visit the American Board of Medical Specialties under Member Boards.

INTERNAL MEDICINE

An **Internist** is a personal physician who provides long-term, comprehensive care in the office and in the hospital, managing both common and complex illnesses of adolescents, adults, and the elderly. Internists are trained in the diagnosis and treatment of cancer, infections and diseases affecting the heart, blood, kidneys, joints, and the digestive, respiratory, and vascular systems. They are also trained in the essentials of primary care internal medicine, which incorporates an understanding of disease prevention, wellness, substance abuse, mental health, and effective treatment of common problems of the eyes, ears, skin, nervous system, and reproductive organs.

Specialty training required prior to Board Certification: 3 years

Subspecialties
To become certified in a particular subspecialty, a physician must be Board Certified by the American Board of Internal Medicine and complete additional training as specified by the Board. The descriptions that follow are of internist specialties.

Adolescent Medicine
An Internist who specializes in Adolescent Medicine is a multidisciplinary health care specialist trained in the unique physical, psychological, and social characteristics of adolescents, their health care problems and needs.

Advanced Heart Failure and Transplant Cardiology
The Heart Failure and Transplant Cardiology internist has the special knowledge and skills required of cardiologists for evaluating and optimally managing patients with heart failure, particularly

patients with advanced heart failure, with devices, including ventricular assist devices, and patients who have undergone or are awaiting transplantation.

Cardiovascular Disease

These internists specialize in diseases of the heart and blood vessels and manage complex cardiac conditions, such as heart attacks and life-threatening, abnormal heartbeat rhythms.

Clinical Cardiac Electrophysiology

This is a field of special interest within the subspecialty of cardiovascular disease, which involves intricate technical procedures to evaluate heart rhythms and determine appropriate treatment.

Critical Care Medicine

An internist trained in Critical Care Medicine has expertise in the diagnosis, treatment, and support of critically ill and injured patients, particularly trauma victims and patients with multiple organ dysfunctions. This physician also coordinates patient care among the primary physician, critical care staff and other specialists.

Endocrinology, Diabetes and Metabolism

This internist concentrates on disorders of the internal (endocrine) glands such as the thyroid and adrenal glands. This specialist also deals with disorders such as diabetes, metabolic and nutritional disorders, obesity, pituitary diseases, and menstrual and sexual problems.

Gastroenterology

A Gastroenterologist specializes in diagnosis and treatment of diseases of the digestive organs, including the stomach, bowels, liver, and gallbladder. This specialist treats conditions such as abdominal pain, ulcers, diarrhea, cancer, and jaundice and performs complex diagnostic and therapeutic procedures using endoscopes to visualize internal organs.

Geriatric Medicine
A Gerontologist is an internist who has special knowledge of the aging process and special skills in the diagnostic, therapeutic, preventive, and rehabilitative aspects of illness in the elderly. This specialist cares for geriatric patients in the patient's home, the office, long-term care settings such as nursing homes and in the hospital.

Hematology
A Hematologist has additional training and specializes in diseases of the blood, spleen and lymph. This specialist treats conditions such as anemia, clotting disorders, sickle cell disease, hemophilia, leukemia, and lymphoma.

Hospice and Palliative Medicine
An internist who has special knowledge and skills to prevent and relieve suffering experienced by patients with life-limiting illnesses, this specialist works with an interdisciplinary hospice or palliative care team to maximize quality of life while addressing the physical, psychological, social, and spiritual needs of both patient and family.

Infectious Disease
These internists deal with infectious diseases of all types and in all organ systems. Conditions requiring selective use of antibiotics call for this special skill. This physician often diagnoses and treats AIDS patients and patients with fevers which have not been explained.

Infectious disease specialists may also have expertise in preventive medicine and travel medicine.

Interventional Cardiology

An area of medicine within the subspecialty of Cardiology that uses specialized imaging and other diagnostic techniques to evaluate blood flow and pressure in the coronary arteries and chambers of the heart and uses technical procedures and medications to treat abnormalities that impair the function of the cardiovascular system.

Medical Oncology

A Medical Oncologist specializes in the diagnosis and treatment of all types of cancer and other benign and malignant tumors. This specialist decides on and administers therapy for these malignancies, as well as consults with surgeons and radiotherapists on other treatments for cancer.

Nephrology

A Nephrologist treats disorders of the kidney, high blood pressure, fluid and mineral balance, and dialysis of body wastes when the kidneys do not function. This specialist consults with surgeons about kidney transplantation.

Pulmonary Disease

A pulmonologist treats diseases of the lungs and airways. He or she diagnoses and treats cancer, pneumonia, pleurisy, asthma, occupational and environmental diseases, bronchitis, sleep disorders, emphysema, and other complex disorders of the lungs.

Rheumatology

Rheumatologists treat diseases of joints, muscle, bones, and tendons. This specialist diagnoses and treats arthritis, back pain, muscle strains, common athletic injuries, and collagen diseases.

Sleep Medicine

Internists specializing in sleep medicine have a demonstrated expertise in the diagnosis and management of clinical conditions that occur during sleep, that disturb sleep, or that are affected by disturbances in the wake-sleep cycle. This specialist is skilled in the analysis and interpretation of comprehensive polysomnography and well-versed in emerging research and management of a sleep laboratory.

Sports Medicine

Sports Medicine internists specialize in preventing, diagnosing, and treating injuries related to participating in sports and/or exercise. In addition to the study of those fields that focus on prevention, diagnosis, treatment and management of injuries, sports medicine also deals with illnesses and diseases that might have effects on health and physical performance.

Transplant Hepatology

Transplant Hepatology internists have the special knowledge and skill required of a Gastroenterologist to care for patients prior to and following hepatic transplantation that spans all phases of liver transplantation. Selection of appropriate recipients requires assessment by a team having experience in evaluating the severity and prognosis of patients with liver disease.

SURGERY (GENERAL SURGERY)

A **General Surgeon** has principal expertise in the diagnosis and care of patients with diseases and disorders affecting the abdomen, digestive tract, endocrine system, breast, skin, and blood vessels. A General Surgeon is also trained in the care of pediatric and cancer patients and in the treatment of patients who are injured or critically ill. Common conditions treated by General Surgeons include hernias, breast tumors, gallstones, appendicitis, pancreatitis, bowel obstructions, colon inflammation and colon cancer. Some General Surgeons pursue additional training and specialize in the fields of Trauma Surgery, Transplant Surgery, Surgical Oncology, Pediatric Surgery, Vascular Surgery, and others.
Specialty training required prior to Board Certification: 5 years

In addition to a general certificate in Surgery (General Surgery), the American Board of Surgery issues a general certificate in Vascular Surgery. A **Vascular Surgeon** has expertise in the diagnosis and care of patients with diseases and disorders affecting the arteries, veins, and lymphatic systems, excluding vessels of the brain and heart. Common procedures performed by vascular surgeons include the opening of artery blockages, repair of veins to improve circulation, treatment of aneurysms (bulges) in the aorta, and care of patients suffering vascular trauma. Vascular Surgeons are also trained in the treatment of vascular disease by medical (non-surgical) means.
Specialty training required prior to Board Certification: 5-7 years

Surgical Subspecialties

To become certified in a particular subspecialty, a physician must be Board Certified by the American Board of Surgery and complete additional training as specified by the Member Board.

General Surgical Oncology

A surgeon trained in complex general surgical oncology has specialized expertise in the diagnosis, multidisciplinary treatment, and rehabilitation of patients with rare, unusual or complex cancers. Typically, these surgeons work in cancer centers or academic institutions and coordinate patient care with other oncologic specialists. They also provide community outreach in cancer prevention and education, as well as lead cancer studies.

Hospice and Palliative Medicine

These surgeons have special knowledge and skills to prevent and relieve the suffering experienced by patients with life-limiting illnesses. They work with an interdisciplinary hospice or palliative care team to maximize quality of life while addressing the physical, psychological, social, and spiritual needs of both patient and family.

Pediatric Surgery

A Pediatric Surgeon is a General Surgeon with specialized training in the diagnosis and care of premature and newborn infants, children, and adolescents. This care includes the detection and correction of fetal abnormalities, repair of birth defects, treatment of injuries in children and adolescents, and the treatment of the pediatric cancer patient, as well as conditions treated in adults by General Surgeons, such as appendicitis, hernias, acid reflux and bowel obstructions.

Surgery of the Hand

A surgeon trained in surgery of the hand has expertise in the surgical, medical, and rehabilitative care of patients with diseases, injuries, and disorders affecting the hand, wrist, and forearm. Common conditions treated by a hand surgeon include carpal tunnel syndrome, trigger fingers, ganglia (lumps), sports injuries to the hand and wrist, and hand injuries involving cut tendons, nerves, and arteries. Hand Surgeons may be General Surgeons, Orthopedic Surgeons or Plastic Surgeons who have received additional training in this area.

Surgical Critical Care

A surgeon trained in Surgical Critical Care has expertise in the diagnosis, treatment, and support of critically ill and injured patients, particularly trauma victims and patients with multiple organ dysfunctions.

There are many, many more subspecialties. To find those, visit the American Board of Medical Specialties-Certification Matters or refer to the resource list at the end of this book.

Last Bit of Advice...

Be your own advocate. It doesn't matter which physician or specialist you choose, go to the doctor's office prepared to communicate your concerns. Doctors go through years of training and experience to build a foundation of knowledge about the human body. They rely on that education and training to help identify diseases and conditions that ail us.

Even though they have compiled all that knowledge, the human body is very complex and unique to each of us. With that in mind, a diagnosis may be delayed while the doctor tries to rule out certain diseases and conditions. The lesson in that: **DON'T GIVE UP**. If something isn't right with your body and the doctor can't find it, that doesn't mean it doesn't exist. Be persistent as the man in the example in Chapter 2 was, until whatever ails you is diagnosed and treated. That mindset could save your life because the doctors are making an educated or experienced guess. Most times they are right. Sometimes they are wrong. Like you, they are very human. And, if you are not satisfied with their results, **GET A SECOND OR THIRD OPINION**.

Medical Records

At the back of this book is a tool to help you organize your thoughts and your records in your effort to find the right doctor. Be able to access your health information easily and quickly and track your medications with these goals in mind.

1) Know the medications you are currently taking, including dosage.
2) Know the medications you took but did not work.
3) Know the medications that trigger allergies.
4) Know which medications react negatively or reduces the effects of other medications. If you don't know, ask. Have the list of your medications available so your doctor will know.
5) Most doctor offices will ask you to update their records with the medications you are taking. Take this list with you to have added to their records to save time.

Medical Record keeping has changed over the years. Hospitals and doctors' offices were mandated to implement the use of electronic medical records by 2017. Incentives from Medicare began in 2011 to help prod doctors toward implementing the keeping of electronic medical records sooner. Healthcare systems and group practices and groups that refer are now providing electronic access to each other's medical records. This practice is improving the delivery and quality of patient care by helping to provide a whole health status of the patient to a treating physician.

In the meantime...

- *Do you have a copy of your medical records?*

- *Have you changed physicians?*

- *Don't remember when you were last immunized? Do you have your immunization records?*

So, if and when you change doctors, don't forget to request a copy of your medical records. Then, take a copy to your new doctor to ensure continuation of care. Make sure you retain a copy of your own records.

Can You Pay?

Whether insured or uninsured, your provider must inform you of a good faith estimate of medical items and services according to the No Surprises Act of 2022. This act also requires health plans to provide a way to appeal certain decisions. The No Surprises Act applies and affects patients receiving care out-of-network as well.

Conclusion

Go one step further. Make your decisions about quality of life and treatment prior to admission to a hospital. Talk to your doctor about your expectations. Have a loved one act on your behalf if you are unable to represent yourself. Their intervention or oversight could create a more collaborative effort to make and keep you healthy. Your decisions can and should be formalized with an Advanced Directive or an Appointment of a Health Care Agent. Check your state or legal adviser for information on the appropriate paperwork and filing.

Pay it forward. Going to the hospital shouldn't be a lone endeavor. Be your friend's or a family member's healthcare advocate. Buddy up and collaborate with their caregivers, too. All in all, our country's healthcare system is very effective. The doctors and nurses that provide healthcare services are dedicated. This book is intended to make you feel comfortable with your healthcare provider by choosing one that meets your needs.

Good

Luck!!!

RESOURCES

State Medical Licensing Entities

Alabama Board of Medical Examiners & Medical Licensure Commission of
Alabama

Alaska State Medical Board

Arizona Medical Board

Arkansas State Medical Board

California Medical Board of California

Colorado Department of Regulatory Agencies

Connecticut Department of Public Health

Delaware Board of Medical Licensure and Discipline

District of Columbia Department of Health

Florida Department of Health

Georgia Composite Medical Board

Hawaii Professional and Vocational Licensing

Idaho Board of Medicine

Illinois Department of Professional and Financial Regulation

Indiana Medical Licensing Board

Iowa Board of Medicine

Kansas Board of Healing Arts

Kentucky Board of Medical Licensure

Louisiana State Board of Medical Examiners

Maine Agency Licenses Management Systems

Maryland Board of Physicians

Massachusetts Department of Public Safety

Michigan Department of Licensing & Regulatory Affairs

Minnesota Board of Medical Practice

Mississippi Board of Medical Licensure

Missouri Division of Professional Registration

Montana Department of Labor and Industry

Nebraska Department of Health and Human Services

Nevada State Board of Medical Examiners

New Hampshire State Board of Medicine

New Jersey Division of Consumer Affairs

New Mexico Regulation and Licensing Department

New York Office of the Professions

North Carolina Medical Board

North Dakota Board of Medical Examiners

Ohio State Medical Board

Oklahoma Board of Medical Licensure and Supervision

Oregon Medical Board

Pennsylvania Bureau of Professional and Occupational Affairs

Rhode Island Board of Medical Licensure and Discipline

South Carolina Department of Labor, Licensing, and Regulation

South Dakota Board of Medical and Osteopathic Examiners

Tennessee Department of Health

Texas Medical Board

Utah Division of Occupational

Vermont Department of Health

Virginia Department of Health Professions

Washington State Department of Health

West Virginia Board of Medicine

Wisconsin Department of Safety and Professional Services

Wyoming Board of Medicine

American Board of Medical Specialties (ABMS)

The American Board of Allergy and Immunology
The American Board of **Anesthesiology**
The American Board of **Colon and Rectal Surgery**
The American Board of **Dermatology**
The American Board of **Emergency Medicine**
The American Board of **Family Medicine**
The American Board of **Internal Medicine**
The American Board of **Medical Genetics**
The American Board of **Neurological Surgery**
The American Board of **Nuclear Medicine**
The American Board of **Obstetrics and Gynecology**
The American Board of **Ophthalmology**
The American Board of **Orthopaedic Surgery**
The American Board of **Otolaryngology**
The American Board of **Pathology**
The American Board of **Pediatrics**
The American Board of **Physical Medicine and Rehabilitation**
The American Board of **Plastic Surgery**
The American Board of **Preventive Medicine**
The American Board of **Psychiatry and Neurology**
The American Board of **Radiology**
The American Board of **Surgery**
The American Board of **Thoracic Surgery**
The American Board of **Urology**

American Osteopathic Association (AOA)

Specialty Certifying Boards

American Osteopathic Board of Anesthesiology (AOBA)

American Osteopathic Board of Dermatology (AOBD)

American Osteopathic Board of Emergency Medicine (AOBEM)

American Osteopathic Board of Family Physicians (AOBFP)

American Osteopathic Board of Internal Medicine (AOBIM)

American Osteopathic Board of Neurology & Psychiatry (AOBNP)

Amer Osteopathic Board of Neuromusculoskeletal Medicine (AOBNMM)

American Osteopathic Board of Nuclear Medicine (AOBNM)

American Osteopathic Board of Obstetrics & Gynecology (AOBOG)

American Osteopathic Board of Ophthalmology & Otolaryngology (AOBOO)

American Osteopathic Board of Orthopedic Surgery (AOBOS)

American Osteopathic Board of Pathology (AOBPa)

American Osteopathic Board of Pediatrics (AOBP)

Amer Osteopathic Board of Physical Medicine & Rehabilitation (AOBPMR)

American Osteopathic Board of Preventive Medicine (AOBPM)

American Osteopathic Board of Proctology (AOBPR)

American Osteopathic Board of Radiology (AOBR)

American Osteopathic Board of Surgery (AOBS)

Criminal Background Checks

County and State Arrest Records
Instant Checkmate
Sentry Link

Other Sources

Checkbook
Doc Boards
Health Grades
US Health News Top Doctors

NOTE: *This is not an endorsement of these products, but examples of tools you can use.*

Related Definitions
and Explanations

Allied Health Professional

Practitioners who may provide health care, dependently requiring supervision or independently without supervision, are considered allied health professionals. There are a variety of health care professions that may fall into this group, usually defined by the organizations for which they work. The most recognized non-physician practitioners who provide healthcare are nurse midwives, CRNA's, nurse practitioners, physician assistants, physical therapists, optometrists, psychologists, and audiologists.

Allopathic Doctor

An allopathic doctor has received a medical degree with the title, MD. Allopaths are trained in conventional medicine and how to combat disease by use of remedies, such as drugs or surgeries.

Board Certified

A physician who is board certified has mastered the highest level of expertise in his or her profession and demonstrates this by passing the board certification exam and maintaining certification through continuous education and training.

Fellowship

Advanced training in a subspecialized area upon completion of the residency program, fellowships may be an additional year or two of the residency on a focused area such as cardiology or thoracic surgery. Or fellowships may be experienced as a hands-on experience within a physician group or hospital program.

Geriatrician

This physician has subspecialized in Geriatrics after training in either Internal Medicine or Family Practice. The focus for this profession is on treating senior adults.

Internship

This is the first year of a residency program, which may be spent in a rotational program to determine whether to pursue a surgical or medicine track.

Nurse Practitioner

A nurse practitioner is a nurse who has completed graduate level education (masters or doctorate). This individual may also have received education and certification in a specialized area such as Family Practice, Pediatrics, Oncology, or Geriatrics. In some states, nurse practitioners may practice independently without physician supervision.

Osteopathic Doctor

An osteopathic doctor has received a medical degree with the title, DO. Osteopaths are trained in preventive medicine with the philosophy to treat the whole patient.

Palliative Care

This specialized medical care is given to people who have a serious illness and focuses on the quality of the patient's life, including the body, mind, and spirit.

Pediatrician

This specialist deals with the medical care of infants, children, and adolescents and, usually, does not see anyone over the age of 18. However, some childhood diseases that may transfer into adulthood may warrant pediatric follow-up.

Physician Assistant

A physician assistant can perform many of the tasks carried out by a supervising or sponsoring physician within the confines of the state's authorization to do so. Their education is modeled after the education of the physician in order to complement the services provided by a physician.

Practitioner

This term is used interchangeably with doctors or allied health professionals. You will see this used in healthcare terminology referring to individuals who provide patient care.

Residency

A medical school graduate receives graduate medical education in a hospital setting to obtain hands-on training while practicing medicine or surgery. These individuals receive in-depth training in any of the primary specialties, such as medicine, family medicine, emergency medicine, anesthesiology, pathology, and more.

Personal Medical and Medication Records Tools

MEDICATION HISTORY HELPER

PATIENT'S NAME: DATE OF BIRTH:
Medication Name:
Dosage: Frequency:
Prescribed by:
Date Prescribed: Last Refill Date:
Drug Interactions:
Medication Name:
Dosage: Frequency:
Prescribed by:
Date Prescribed: Last Refill Date:
Drug Interactions:
Medication Name:
Dosage: Frequency:
Prescribed by:
Date Prescribed: Last Refill Date:
Drug Interactions:
NOTES:

MEDICATION HISTORY HELPER/ 2

PATIENT'S NAME: DATE OF BIRTH:
Medication Name:
Dosage: Frequency:
Prescribed by:
Date Prescribed: Last Refill Date:
Drug Interactions:
Medication Name:
Dosage: Frequency:
Prescribed by:
Date Prescribed: Last Refill Date:
Drug Interactions:
Medication Name:
Dosage: Frequency:
Prescribed by:
Date Prescribed: Last Refill Date:
Drug Interactions:
NOTES:

MEDICATION HISTORY HELPER/ 3

PATIENT'S NAME: DATE OF BIRTH:
Medication Name:
Dosage: Frequency:
Prescribed by:
Date Prescribed: Last Refill Date:
Drug Interactions:
Medication Name:
Dosage: Frequency:
Prescribed by:
Date Prescribed: Last Refill Date:
Drug Interactions:
Medication Name:
Dosage: Frequency:
Prescribed by:
Date Prescribed: Last Refill Date:
Drug Interactions:
NOTES:

MEDICATION HISTORY HELPER/ 4

PATIENT'S NAME: DATE OF BIRTH:
Medication Name:
Dosage: Frequency:
Prescribed by:
Date Prescribed: Last Refill Date:
Drug Interactions:
Medication Name:
Dosage: Frequency:
Prescribed by:
Date Prescribed: Last Refill Date:
Drug Interactions:
Medication Name:
Dosage: Frequency:
Prescribed by:
Date Prescribed: Last Refill Date:
Drug Interactions:
NOTES:

PERSONAL PHYSICIAN(S) DIRECTORY

Doctor's Name:
Group Name:
Doctor Type:
Last Visit: Next Scheduled Visit/Time:
Office Location:
Telephone: Fax:
Email:
Lab Work Date:
EKG/X-Ray Date:
Date Obtained Final Copy of Medical Records:
NOTES:

PERSONAL PHYSICIAN(S) DIRECTORY/ 2

Doctor's Name:
Group Name:
Doctor Type:
Last Visit: Next Scheduled Visit/Time:
Office Location:
Telephone: Fax:
Email:
Lab Work Date:
EKG/X-Ray Date:
Date Obtained Final Copy of Medical Records:
NOTES:

PERSONAL PHYSICIAN(S) DIRECTORY/ 3

Doctor's Name:
Group Name:
Doctor Type:
Last Visit: Next Scheduled Visit/Time:
Office Location:
Telephone: Fax:
Email:
Lab Work Date:
EKG/X-Ray Date:
Date Obtained Final Copy of Medical Records:
NOTES:

PERSONAL MEDICAL INFORMATION

PATIENT'S NAME: DATE OF BIRTH:
Health Care Plan:
Health Care Plan ID: Group ID:
Drug Allergies:
Blood Type:
Chronic Conditions:
Preferred Hospital/Location:
Emergency Contact Name:
Emergency Contact Number:
Power of Attorney/Executor of Living Will:
Executor Contact Info/Number:
NOTES:

PERSONAL MEDICAL INFORMATION-2

Health Care Plan:
Health Care Plan ID: Group ID:
Drug Allergies:
Blood Type:
Chronic Conditions:
Preferred Hospital/Location:
Emergency Contact Name:
Emergency Contact Number:
Power of Attorney/Executor of Living Will:
Executor Contact Info/Number:
NOTES:

IMMUNIZATION CHECKLIST

PATIENT'S NAME: DATE OF BIRTH:	
IMMUNIZATION TYPE	**DATE(s)**
Chicken Pox (varicella)	
Diphtheria and Tetanus Toxoids and acellular Pertussis (DTaP)	
Flu	
Hepatitis A	
Hepatitis B	
Human Papillomavirus (HPV)	
Meningococcal	
MMR (Measles, Mumps, Rubella)	
Pneumococcal	
Polio	
Rotavirus	
Tetanus	
Zoster	

DOCTOR FINDERS JOURNAL

DOCTOR FINDERS JOURNAL/ 5

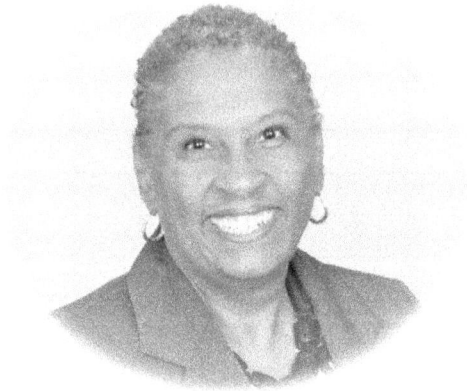

Dilsa S. Bailey is a writer, speaker, and consultant with over 30 years of experience in professional healthcare credentialing. She has worked in hospitals and managed care organizations, ranging from the academic to commercial and from Medicare to Medicaid. Her work has assisted those organizations' clinical leadership, affiliating or hiring thousands of doctors. For more information about her profession, visit www.therightcredentials.com. Reach out to Dilsa to have her speak at your next Health and Wellness Event.

YOUR NOTES

YOUR NOTES

www.ingramcontent.com/pod-product-compliance
Lightning Source LLC
Chambersburg PA
CBHW031220290326
41931CB00035B/622